DATE DUE

JA 0 2 '17

Cause ——— Treat-
ments, ——— dition -

PRINTED IN U.S.A.

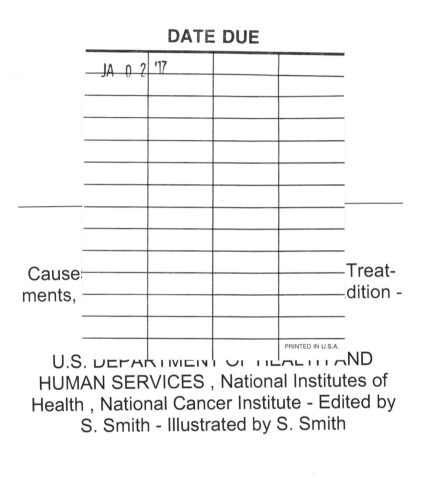

U.S. DEPARTMENT OF HEALTH AND
HUMAN SERVICES , National Institutes of
Health , National Cancer Institute - Edited by
S. Smith - Illustrated by S. Smith

Leukemia

Table of Contents

About This Booklet

This National Cancer Institute (NCI) booklet (NIH Publication No. 08-3775) is about leukemia,* cancer that starts in the tissue that forms blood. Each year in the United States, more than 40,800 adults and 3,500 children learn they have this disease.

Learning about medical care for leukemia can help you take an active part in making choices about your care. This booklet tells about:

Diagnosis
Treatment options
Supportive care you may need before, during, or after treatment
Tests the doctor may give you during follow-up visits
Taking part in research studies
This booklet has lists of questions that you may want to ask your doctor. Many people find it helpful to take a list of questions to a doctor visit. To help remember what your doctor says, you can take notes or ask whether you may use a tape recorder. You may also want to have a family member or friend go with you when you talk with the doctor -- to take notes, ask questions, or just to listen.

What Is Leukemia?

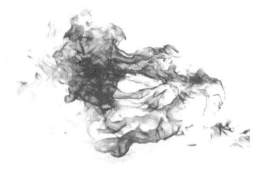

Leukemia is cancer that starts in the tissue that forms blood. To understand cancer, it helps to know how normal blood cells form.

Normal Blood Cells

Most blood cells develop from cells in the bone marrow called stem cells. Bone marrow is the soft material in the center of most bones.

Stem cells mature into different kinds of blood cells. Each kind has a special job:

White blood cells help fight infection. There are several types of white blood cells.

Red blood cells carry oxygen to tissues throughout the body.

Platelets help form blood clots that control bleeding.

White blood cells, red blood cells, and platelets are made from stem cells as the body needs them. When cells grow old or get damaged, they die, and new cells take their place.

First, a stem cell matures into either a myeloid stem cell or a lymphoid stem cell:

A myeloid stem cell matures into a myeloid blast. The blast can form a red blood cell, platelets, or one of several types of white blood cells.

A lymphoid stem cell matures into a lymphoid blast. The blast can form one of several types of white blood cells, such as B cells or T cells.

The white blood cells that form from myeloid blasts are different from the white blood cells that form from lymphoid blasts.

Most blood cells mature in the bone marrow and then move into the blood vessels. Blood flowing through the blood vessels and heart is called the peripheral blood.

Leukemia Cells

What Is Leukemia?

In a person with leukemia, the bone marrow makes abnormal white blood cells. The abnormal cells are leukemia cells.

Unlike normal blood cells, leukemia cells don't die when they should. They may crowd out normal white blood cells, red blood cells, and platelets. This makes it hard for normal blood cells to do their work.

Types of Leukemia

The types of leukemia can be grouped based on how quickly the disease develops and gets worse. Leukemia is either chronic (which usually gets worse slowly) or acute (which usually gets worse quickly):

Chronic leukemia: Early in the disease, the leukemia cells can still do some of the work of normal white blood cells. People may not have any symptoms at first. Doctors often find chronic leukemia during a routine checkup - before there are any symptoms. Slowly, chronic leukemia gets worse. As the number of leukemia cells in the blood increases, people get symptoms, such as swollen lymph nodes or infections. When symptoms do appear, they are usually mild at first and get worse gradually.

Acute leukemia: The leukemia cells can't do any of the work of normal white blood cells. The number of leukemia cells increases rapidly. Acute leukemia usually worsens quickly.

The types of leukemia also can be grouped based on the type of white blood cell that is affected. Leukemia can start in lymphoid cells or myeloid cells. See the picture of these cells. Leukemia that affects lymphoid cells is called lymphoid, lymphocytic, or lymphoblastic leukemia. Leukemia that affects myeloid cells is called myeloid, myelogenous, or myeloblastic leukemia.

Leukemia

There are four common types of leukemia:

Chronic lymphocytic leukemia (CLL): CLL affects lymphoid cells and usually grows slowly. It accounts for more than 15,000 new cases of leukemia each year. Most often, people diagnosed with the disease are over age 55. It almost never affects children.

Chronic myeloid leukemia (CML): CML affects myeloid cells and usually grows slowly at first. It accounts for nearly 5,000 new cases of leukemia each year. It mainly affects adults.

Acute lymphocytic (lymphoblastic) leukemia (ALL): ALL affects lymphoid cells and grows quickly. It accounts for more than 5,000 new cases of leukemia each year. ALL is the most common type of leukemia in young children. It also affects adults.

Acute myeloid leukemia (AML): AML affects myeloid cells and grows quickly. It accounts for more than 13,000 new cases of leukemia each year. It occurs in both adults and children.

Hairy cell leukemia is a rare type of chronic leukemia. This booklet is not about hairy cell leukemia or other rare types of leukemia. Together, these rare leukemias account for fewer than 6,000 new cases of leukemia each year. The Cancer Information Service (1-800-4-CANCER) can provide information about rare types of leukemia.

Risk Factors

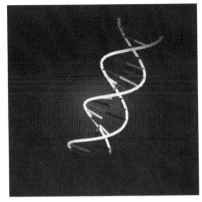

When you're told that you have cancer, it's natural to wonder what may have caused the disease. No one knows the exact causes of leukemia. Doctors seldom know why one person gets leukemia and another doesn't. However, research shows that certain risk factors increase the chance that a person will get this disease.

The risk factors may be different for the different types of leukemia:

Radiation: People exposed to very high levels of radiation are much more likely than others to get acute myeloid leukemia, chronic myeloid leukemia, or acute lymphocytic leukemia.

Atomic bomb explosions: Very high levels of radiation have been caused by atomic bomb explosions (such as those in Japan during World War II). People, especially children, who survive atomic bomb explosions are at increased risk of leukemia.

Radiation therapy: Another source of exposure to high levels of radiation is medical treatment for cancer and other conditions. Radiation therapy can increase the risk of leukemia.

Diagnostic x-rays: Dental x-rays and other diagnostic x-rays (such as CT scans) expose people to much lower levels of radiation. It's not known yet whether this low level of radiation to children or adults is linked to leukemia. Researchers are studying whether having many x-rays may increase the risk of leukemia. They are also studying whether CT scans during childhood are linked with increased risk of developing leukemia.

Smoking: Smoking cigarettes increases the risk of acute myeloid leukemia.

Benzene: Exposure to benzene in the workplace can cause acute myeloid leukemia. It may also cause chronic myeloid leukemia or acute lymphocytic leukemia. Benzene is used widely in the chemical industry. It's also found in cigarette smoke and gasoline.

Chemotherapy: Cancer patients treated with certain types of cancer-fighting drugs sometimes later get acute myeloid leukemia or acute lymphocytic leukemia. For example, being treated with drugs known as alkylating agents or topoisomerase inhibitors is linked with a small chance of later developing acute leukemia.

Down syndrome and certain other inherited diseases: Down syndrome and certain other inherited diseases increase the risk of developing acute leukemia.

Myelodysplastic syndrome and certain other blood disorders: People with certain blood disorders are at increased risk of acute myeloid leukemia.

Human T-cell leukemia virus type I (HTLV-I): People with HTLV-I infection are at increased risk of a rare type of leukemia known as adult T-cell leukemia. Although the HTLV-I virus may cause this rare disease, adult T-cell leukemia and other types of leukemia are not contagious.

Family history of leukemia: It's rare for more than one person in a family to have leukemia. When it does happen, it's most likely to involve chronic lymphocytic leukemia. However, only a few people with chronic lymphocytic leukemia have a father, mother, brother, sister, or child who also has the disease.

Having one or more risk factors does not mean that a person will get leukemia. Most people who have risk factors never develop the disease.

Symptoms

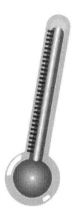

Like all blood cells, leukemia cells travel through the body. The symptoms of leukemia depend on the number of leukemia cells and where these cells collect in the body.

People with chronic leukemia may not have symptoms. The doctor may find the disease during a routine blood test.

People with acute leukemia usually go to their doctor because they feel sick. If the brain is affected, they may have headaches, vomiting, confusion, loss of muscle control, or seizures. Leukemia also can affect other parts of the body such as the digestive tract, kidneys, lungs, heart, or testes.

Common symptoms of chronic or acute leukemia may include:

• Swollen lymph nodes that usually don't hurt (especially lymph nodes in the neck or armpit)
• Fevers or night sweats
• Frequent infections
• Feeling weak or tired
• Bleeding and bruising easily (bleeding gums, purplish patches in the skin, or tiny red spots under the skin)
• Swelling or discomfort in the abdomen (from a swollen spleen or liver)
• Weight loss for no known reason
• Pain in the bones or joints

Most often, these symptoms are not due to cancer. An infection or other health problems may also cause these symptoms. Only a doctor can tell for sure.

Anyone with these symptoms should tell the doctor so that problems can be diagnosed and treated as early as possible.

Diagnosis

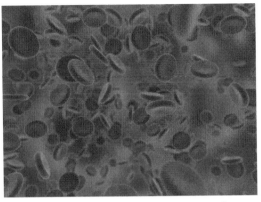

Doctors sometimes find leukemia after a routine blood test. If you have symptoms that suggest leukemia, your doctor will try to find out what's causing the problems. Your doctor may ask about your personal and family medical history.

You may have one or more of the following tests:

Physical exam: Your doctor checks for swollen lymph nodes, spleen, or liver.

Blood tests: The lab does a complete blood count to check the number of white blood cells, red blood cells, and platelets. Leukemia causes a very high level of white blood cells. It may also cause low levels of platelets and hemoglobin, which is found inside red blood cells.

Biopsy: Your doctor removes tissue to look for cancer cells. A biopsy is the only sure way to know whether leukemia cells are in your bone marrow. Before the sample is taken, local anesthesia is used to numb the area. This helps reduce the pain. Your doctor removes some bone marrow from your hipbone or another large bone. A pathologist uses a microscope to check the tissue for leukemia cells. There are two ways your doctor can obtain bone marrow. Some people will have both procedures during the same visit:

Bone marrow aspiration: The doctor uses a thick, hollow needle to remove samples of bone marrow.

Bone marrow biopsy: The doctor uses a very thick, hollow needle to remove a small piece of bone and bone marrow.

Other Tests

The tests that your doctor orders for you depend on your symptoms and type of leukemia. You may have other tests:

Cytogenetics: The lab looks at the chromosomes of cells from samples of blood, bone marrow, or lymph nodes. If abnormal chromosomes are found, the test can show what type of leukemia you have. For example, people with CML have an abnormal chromosome called the Philadelphia chromosome.

Spinal tap: Your doctor may remove some of the cerebrospinal fluid (the fluid that fills the spaces in and around the brain and spinal cord). The doctor uses a long, thin needle to remove fluid from the lower spine. The procedure takes about 30 minutes and is performed with local anesthesia. You must lie flat for several hours afterward to keep from getting a headache. The lab checks the fluid for leukemia cells or other signs of problems.

Chest x-ray: An x-ray can show swollen lymph nodes or other signs of disease in your chest.

You may want to ask your doctor these questions before having a bone marrow aspiration or biopsy:

• Will you remove the sample of bone marrow from the hip or from another bone?

• Where will I go for this procedure?

• Will I have to do anything to prepare for it?

• How long will it take? Will I be awake?

• Will it hurt? What will you do to prevent or control the pain?

• Are there any risks? What are the chances of infection or bleeding after the procedure?

• How long will it take me to recover?

• How soon will I know the results? Who will explain them to me?

• If I do have leukemia, who will talk to me about next steps? When?

Treatment

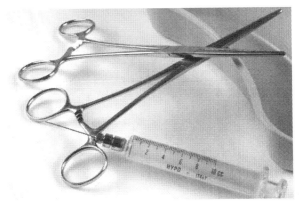

People with leukemia have many treatment options. The options are watchful waiting, chemotherapy, targeted therapy, biological therapy, radiation therapy, and stem cell transplant. If your spleen is enlarged, your doctor may suggest surgery to remove it. Sometimes a combination of these treatments is used.

The choice of treatment depends mainly on the following:

- The type of leukemia (acute or chronic)
- Your age
- Whether leukemia cells were found in your cerebrospinal fluid

It also may depend on certain features of the leukemia cells. Your doctor also considers your symptoms and general health.

People with acute leukemia need to be treated right away. The goal of treatment is to destroy signs of leukemia in the body and make symptoms go away. This is called a remission. After people go into remission, more therapy may be given to prevent a relapse. This type of therapy is called consolidation therapy or maintenance therapy. Many people with acute leukemia can be cured.

If you have chronic leukemia without symptoms, you may not need cancer treatment right away. Your doctor will watch your health closely so that treatment can start when you begin to have symptoms. Not getting cancer treatment right away is called watchful waiting.

When treatment for chronic leukemia is needed, it can often control the disease and its symptoms. People may receive maintenance therapy to help keep the cancer in remission, but chronic leukemia can seldom be cured with chemotherapy. However, stem cell transplants offer some people with chronic leukemia the chance for cure.

Your doctor can describe your treatment choices, the expected results, and the possible side effects. You and your doctor can work together to develop a treatment plan that meets your medical and personal needs.

You may want to talk with your doctor about taking part in a clinical trial, a research study of new treatment methods. See the Taking Part in Cancer Research section.

Your doctor may refer you to a specialist, or you may ask for a referral. Specialists who treat leukemia include hematologists, medical oncologists, and radiation oncologists. Pediatric oncologists and hematologists treat childhood leukemia. Your health care team may also include an oncology nurse and a registered dietitian.

Whenever possible, people should be treated at a medical center that has doctors experienced in treating leukemia. If this isn't possible, your doctor may discuss the treatment plan with a specialist at such a center.

Before treatment starts, ask your health care team to explain possible side effects and how treatment may change your normal activities. Because cancer treatments often damage healthy cells and tissues, side effects are common. Side effects may not be the same for each person, and they may change from one treatment session to the next.

You may want to ask your doctor these questions before you begin treatment:

- What type of leukemia do I have? How do I get a copy of the report from the pathologist?
- What are my treatment choices? Which do you recommend for me? Why?
- Will I have more than one kind of treatment? How will my treatment change over time?
- What are the expected benefits of each kind of treatment?
- What are the risks and possible side effects of each treatment? What can we do to control the side effects?
- What can I do to prepare for treatment?
- Will I need to stay in the hospital? If so, for how long?
- What is the treatment likely to cost? Will my insurance cover the cost?
- How will treatment affect my normal activities?
- Would a clinical trial be right for me? Can you help me find one?
- How often should I have checkups?

Watchful Waiting

People with chronic lymphocytic leukemia who do not have symptoms may be able to put off having cancer treatment. By delaying treatment, they can avoid the side effects of treatment until they have symptoms.

If you and your doctor agree that watchful waiting is a good idea, you'll have regular checkups (such as every 3 months). You can start treatment if symptoms occur.

Although watchful waiting avoids or delays the side effects of cancer treatment, this choice has risks. It may reduce the chance to control leukemia before it gets worse.

You may decide against watchful waiting if you don't want to live with an untreated leukemia. Some people choose to treat the cancer right away.

If you choose watchful waiting but grow concerned later, you should discuss your feelings with your doctor. A different approach is nearly always available.

You may want to ask your doctor these questions before choosing watchful waiting:
• If I choose watchful waiting, can I change my mind later on?
• Will the leukemia be harder to treat later?
• How often will I have checkups?
• Between checkups, what problems should I report?
Chemotherapy

Many people with leukemia are treated with chemotherapy. Chemotherapy uses drugs to destroy leukemia cells.

Depending on the type of leukemia, you may receive a single drug or a combination of two or more drugs.

You may receive chemotherapy in several different ways:

• By mouth: Some drugs are pills that you can swallow.

• Into a vein (IV): The drug is given through a needle or tube inserted into a vein.

• Through a catheter (a thin, flexible tube): The tube is placed in a large vein, often in the upper chest. A tube that stays in place is useful for patients who need many IV treatments. The health care professional injects drugs into the catheter, rather than directly into a vein. This method avoids the need for many injections, which can cause discomfort and injure the veins and skin.

• Into the cerebrospinal fluid: If the pathologist finds leukemia cells in the fluid that fills the spaces in and around the brain and spinal cord, the doctor may order intrathecal chemotherapy. The doctor injects drugs directly into the cerebrospinal fluid. Intrathecal chemotherapy is given in two ways:

• Into the spinal fluid: The doctor injects the drugs into the spinal fluid.

• Under the scalp: Children and some adult patients receive chemotherapy through a special catheter called an Ommaya reservoir. The doctor places the catheter under the scalp.

The doctor injects the drugs into the catheter. This method avoids the pain of injections into the spinal fluid.

• Intrathecal chemotherapy is used because many drugs given by IV or taken by mouth can't pass through the tightly packed blood vessel walls found in the brain and spinal cord. This network of blood vessels is known as the blood-brain barrier.

Chemotherapy is usually given in cycles. Each cycle has a treatment period followed by a rest period.

You may have your treatment in a clinic, at the doctor's office, or at home. Some people may need to stay in the hospital for treatment.

The side effects depend mainly on which drugs are given and how much. Chemotherapy kills fast-growing leukemia cells, but the drug can also harm normal cells that divide rapidly:

Blood cells: When chemotherapy lowers the levels of healthy blood cells, you're more likely to get infections, bruise or bleed easily, and feel very weak and tired. You'll get blood tests to check for low levels of blood cells. If your levels are low, your health care team may stop the chemotherapy for a while or reduce the dose of drug. There also are medicines that can help your body make new blood cells. Or, you may need a blood transfusion.

Cells in hair roots: Chemotherapy may cause hair loss. If you lose your hair, it will grow back, but it may be somewhat different in color and texture.

Cells that line the digestive tract: Chemotherapy can cause poor appetite, nausea and vomiting, diarrhea, or mouth and lip sores. Ask your health care team about medicines and other ways to help you cope with these problems.

Sperm or egg cells: Some types of chemotherapy can cause infertility.

Children: Most children treated for leukemia appear to have normal fertility when they grow up. However, depending on the drugs and doses used and the age of the patient, some boys and girls may be infertile as adults.

Adult men: Chemotherapy may damage sperm cells. Men may stop making sperm. Because these changes to sperm may be permanent, some men have their sperm frozen and stored before treatment (sperm banking).

Adult women: Chemotherapy may damage the ovaries. Women may have irregular menstrual periods or periods may stop altogether. Women may have symptoms of menopause, such as hot flashes and vaginal dryness. Women who may want to get pregnant in the future should ask their health care team about ways to preserve their eggs before treatment starts.

You may find it helpful to read NCI's booklet Chemotherapy and You.

Targeted Therapy

People with chronic myeloid leukemia and some with acute lymphoblastic leukemia may receive drugs called targeted therapy. Imatinib (Gleevec) tablets were the first targeted therapy approved for chronic myeloid leukemia. Other targeted therapy drugs are now used too.

Targeted therapies use drugs that block the growth of leukemia cells. For example, a targeted therapy may block the action of an abnormal protein that stimulates the growth of leukemia cells.

Side effects include swelling, bloating, and sudden weight gain. Targeted therapy can also cause anemia, nausea, vomiting, diarrhea, muscle cramps, or a rash. Your health care team will monitor you for signs of problems.

You may want to read the NCI fact sheet Targeted Cancer Therapies.

Biological Therapy

Some people with leukemia receive drugs called biological therapy. Biological therapy for leukemia is treatment that improves the body's natural defenses against the disease.

One type of biological therapy is a substance called a monoclonal antibody. It's given by IV infusion. This substance binds to the leukemia cells. One kind of monoclonal antibody carries a toxin that kills the leukemia cells. Another kind helps the immune system destroy leukemia cells.

For some people with chronic myeloid leukemia, the biological therapy is a drug called interferon. It is injected under the skin or into a muscle. It can slow the growth of leukemia cells.

You may have your treatment in a clinic, at the doctor's office, or in the hospital. Other drugs may be given at the same time to prevent side effects.

The side effects of biological therapy differ with the types of substances used, and from person to person. Biological therapies commonly cause a rash or swelling where the drug is injected. They also may cause a headache, muscle aches, a fever, or weakness. Your health care team may check your blood for signs of anemia and other problems.

You may find it helpful to read NCI's booklet Biological Therapy.

You may want to ask your doctor these questions before having chemotherapy, targeted therapy, or biological therapy:

• Which drugs will I get? What will the treatment do?

• Should I see my dentist before treatment begins?

• When will treatment start? When will it end? How often will I have treatments?

• Where will I go for treatment? Will I have to stay in the hospital?

• What can I do to take care of myself during treatment?

• How will we know the treatment is working?

• Will I have side effects during treatment? What side effects should I tell you about? Can I prevent or treat any of these side effects?

• Can these drugs cause side effects later on?

• How often will I need checkups?

Radiation Therapy

Radiation therapy (also called radiotherapy) uses high-energy rays to kill leukemia cells. People receive radiation therapy at a hospital or clinic.

Some people receive radiation from a large machine that is aimed at the spleen, the brain, or other parts of the body where leukemia cells have collected. This type of therapy takes place 5 days a week for several weeks. Others may receive radiation that is directed to the whole body. The radiation treatments are given once or twice a day for a few days, usually before a stem cell transplant.

The side effects of radiation therapy depend mainly on the dose of radiation and the part of the body that is treated. For example, radiation to your abdomen can cause nausea, vomiting, and diarrhea. In addition, your skin in the area being treated may become red, dry, and tender. You also may lose your hair in the treated area.

You are likely to be very tired during radiation therapy, especially after several weeks of treatment. Resting is important, but doctors usually advise patients to try to stay as active as they can.

Although the side effects of radiation therapy can be distressing, they can usually be treated or controlled. You can talk with your doctor about ways to ease these problems.

It may also help to know that, in most cases, the side effects are not permanent. However, you may want to discuss with your doctor the possible long-term effects of radiation treatment.

You may find it helpful to read NCI's booklet Radiation Therapy and You.

You may want to ask your doctor these questions before having radiation therapy:
• Why do I need this treatment?

- When will the treatments begin? How often will they be given? When will they end?
- How will I feel during treatment? Will I be able to continue my normal activities during treatment?
- Will there be side effects? How long will they last?
- Can radiation therapy cause side effects later on?
- What can I do to take care of myself during treatment?
- How will we know if the radiation treatment is working?
- How often will I need checkups?

Stem Cell Transplant

Some people with leukemia receive a stem cell transplant. A stem cell transplant allows you to be treated with high doses of drugs, radiation, or both. The high doses destroy both leukemia cells and normal blood cells in the bone marrow. After you receive highdose chemotherapy, radiation therapy, or both, you receive healthy stem cells through a large vein. (It's like getting a blood transfusion.) New blood cells develop from the transplanted stem cells. The new blood cells replace the ones that were destroyed by treatment.

Stem cell transplants take place in the hospital. Stem cells may come from you or from someone who donates their stem cells to you:

From you: An autologous stem cell transplant uses your own stem cells. Before you get the high-dose chemotherapy or radiation therapy, your stem cells are removed. The cells may be treated to kill any leukemia cells present. Your stem cells are frozen and stored. After you receive high-dose chemotherapy or radiation therapy, the stored stem cells are thawed and returned to you.

From a family member or other donor: An allogeneic stem cell transplant uses healthy stem cells from a donor. Your brother, sister, or parent may be the donor. Sometimes the stem cells come from a donor who isn't related. Doctors use blood tests to learn how closely a donor's cells match your cells.

From your identical twin: If you have an identical twin, a syngeneic stem cell transplant uses stem cells from your healthy twin.

Stem cells come from a few sources. The stem cells usually come from the blood (peripheral stem cell transplant). Or they can come from the bone marrow (bone marrow transplant). Another source of stem cells is umbilical cord blood. Cord blood is taken from a newborn baby and stored in a freezer. When a person gets cord blood, it's called an umbilical cord blood transplant.

After a stem cell transplant, you may stay in the hospital for several weeks or months. You'll be at risk for infections and bleeding because of the large doses of chemotherapy or radiation you received. In time, the transplanted stem cells will begin to produce healthy blood cells.

Another problem is that graft-versus-host disease (GVHD) may occur in people who receive donated stem cells. In GVHD, the donated white blood cells in the stem cell graft react against the patient's normal tissues. Most often, the liver, skin, or digestive tract is affected. GVHD can be mild or very severe. It can occur any time after the transplant, even years later. Steroids or other drugs may help.

You may find it helpful to read NCI's fact sheet Bone Marrow Transplantation and Peripheral Blood Stem Cell Transplantation.

You may want to ask your doctor these questions before having a stem cell transplant:

• What kind of stem cell transplant will I have? If I need a donor, how will we find one?

• How long will I be in the hospital? Will I need special care? How will I be protected from germs? Will my visitors have to wear a mask? Will I?

• What care will I need when I leave the hospital?

• How will we know if the treatment is working?

• What are the risks and the side effects? What can we do about them?

• What changes in normal activities will be necessary?

- What is my chance of a full recovery? How long will that take?
- How often will I need checkups?

Second Opinion

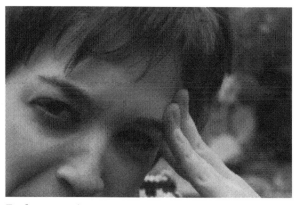

Before starting treatment, you might want a second opinion about your diagnosis and treatment plan. Some people worry that the doctor will be offended if they ask for a second opinion. Usually the opposite is true. Most doctors welcome a second opinion. And many health insurance companies will pay for a second opinion if you or your doctor requests it.

If you get a second opinion, the doctor may agree with your first doctor's diagnosis and treatment plan. Or the second doctor may suggest another approach. Either way, you have more information and perhaps a greater sense of control. You can feel more confident about the decisions you make, knowing that you've looked at your options.

It may take some time and effort to gather your medical records and see another doctor. In most cases, it's not a problem to take several weeks to get a second opinion. The delay in starting treatment usually won't make treatment less effective. To make sure, you should discuss this delay with your doctor. Some people with leukemia need treatment right away.

There are many ways to find a doctor for a second opinion. You can ask your doctor, a local or state medical society, a nearby hospital, or a medical school for names of specialists. NCI's Cancer Information Service at 1-800-4-CANCER can tell you about nearby treatment centers. Other sources can be found in NCI's fact sheet How To Find a Doctor or Treatment Facility If You Have Cancer.

Nonprofit groups with an interest in leukemia may be of help. Many such groups are listed in NCI's database National Organizations That Offer Cancer-Related Services.

Supportive Care

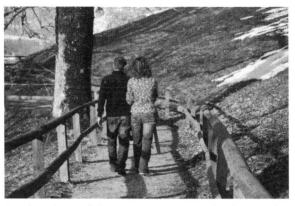

Leukemia and its treatment can lead to other health problems. You can have supportive care before, during, or after cancer treatment.

Supportive care is treatment to prevent or fight infections, to control pain and other symptoms, to relieve the side effects of therapy, and to help you cope with the feelings that a diagnosis of cancer can bring. You may receive supportive care to prevent or control these problems and to improve your comfort and quality of life during treatment.

Infections: Because people with leukemia get infections very easily, you may receive antibiotics and other drugs. Some people receive vaccines against the flu and pneumonia. The health care team may advise you to stay away from crowds and from people with colds and other contagious diseases. If an infection develops, it can be serious and should be treated promptly. You may need to stay in the hospital for treatment.

Anemia and bleeding: Anemia and bleeding are other problems that often require supportive care. You may need a transfusion of red blood cells or platelets. Transfusions help treat anemia and reduce the risk of serious bleeding.

Dental problems: Leukemia and chemotherapy can make the mouth sensitive, easily infected, and likely to bleed. Doctors often advise patients to have a complete dental exam and, if possible, undergo needed dental care before chemotherapy begins. Dentists show patients how to keep their mouth clean and healthy during treatment.

You can get information about supportive care on NCI's Web site at http://www.cancer.gov/cancerinfo/coping and from NCI's Cancer Information Service at 1-800-4-CANCER or LiveHelp (http://www.cancer.gov/livehelp).

Nutrition and Physical Activity

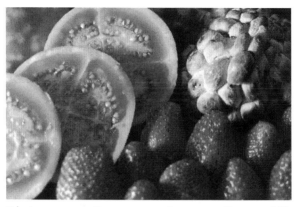

It's important for you to take care of yourself by eating well and staying as active as you can.

You need the right amount of calories to maintain a good weight. You also need enough protein to keep up your strength. Eating well may help you feel better and have more energy.

Sometimes, especially during or soon after treatment, you may not feel like eating. You may be uncomfortable or tired. You may find that foods do not taste as good as they used to. In addition, the side effects of treatment (such as poor appetite, nausea, vomiting, or mouth sores) can make it hard to eat well. Your doctor, a registered dietitian, or another health care provider can suggest ways to deal with these problems.

Also, the NCI booklet Eating Hints has many useful ideas and recipes.

Research shows that people with cancer feel better when they are active. Walking, yoga, and other activities can keep you strong and increase your energy. Exercise may reduce nausea and pain and make treatment easier to handle. It also can help relieve stress. Whatever physical activity you choose, be sure to talk to your doctor before you start. Also, if your activity causes you pain or other problems, be sure to let your doctor or nurse know about it.

Follow-up Care

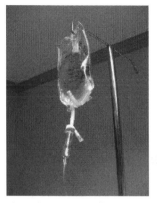

You'll need regular checkups after treatment for leukemia. Checkups help ensure that any changes in your health are noted and treated if needed. If you have any health problems between checkups, you should contact your doctor.

Your doctor will check for return of the cancer. Even when the cancer seems to be completely destroyed, the disease sometimes returns because undetected leukemia cells remained somewhere in your body after treatment. Also, checkups help detect health problems that can result from cancer treatment.

Checkups may include a careful physical exam, blood tests, cytogenetics, x-rays, bone marrow aspiration, or spinal tap.

The NCI has publications to help answer questions about follow-up care and other concerns. You may find it helpful to read the NCI booklet Facing Forward: Life After Cancer Treatment. You may also want to read the NCI fact sheet Follow-up Care After Cancer Treatment.

• You may want to ask your doctor these questions after you have finished treatment:
    • How often will I need checkups?
    • Which follow-up tests do you suggest for me?
    • Between checkups, what health problems or symptoms should I tell you about?

Sources of Support

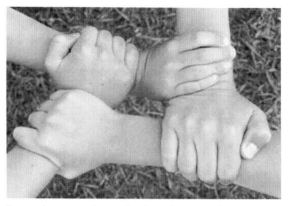

Learning you have leukemia can change your life and the lives of those close to you. These changes can be hard to handle. It's normal for you, your family, and your friends to have new and confusing feelings to work through.

Concerns about treatments and managing side effects, hospital stays, and medical bills are common. You may also worry about caring for your family, keeping your job, or continuing daily activities.

Here's where you can go for support:

Doctors, nurses, and other members of your health care team can answer many of your questions about treatment, working, or other activities.

Social workers, counselors, or members of the clergy can be helpful if you want to talk about your feelings or concerns. Often, social workers can suggest resources for financial aid, transportation, home care, or emotional support.

Support groups can also help. In these groups, patients or their family members meet with other patients or their families to share what they have learned about coping with the disease and the effects of treatment. Groups may offer support in person, over the telephone, or on the Internet. You may want to talk with a member of your health care team about finding a support group.

Information specialists at 1-800-4-CANCER and at LiveHelp (http://www.cancer.gov/livehelp) can help you locate programs, services, and publications. They can give you names of national organizations that offer services to people with cancer and their families.

For tips on coping, you may want to read the NCI booklet Taking Time: Support for People With Cancer.

Taking Part in Cancer Research

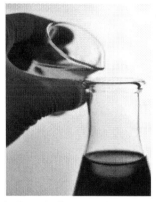

Cancer research has led to real progress in leukemia treatment. Because of research, adults and children with leukemia can look forward to a better quality of life and less chance of dying from the disease. Continuing research offers hope that, in the future, even more people with this disease will be treated successfully.

Doctors all over the country are conducting many types of clinical trials (research studies in which people volunteer to take part). Clinical trials are designed to answer important questions and to find out whether new approaches are safe and effective.

Doctors are studying methods of new and better ways to treat leukemia, and ways to improve quality of life. They are testing new targeted therapy, biological therapy, and chemotherapy. They also are working with various combinations of treatments.

Even if people in a trial do not benefit directly, they still make an important contribution by helping doctors learn more about leukemia and how to control it. Although clinical trials may pose some risks, doctors do all they can to protect their patients.

If you are interested in being part of a clinical trial, talk with your doctor. You may want to read the NCI booklet Taking Part in Cancer Treatment Research Studies. This booklet describes how treatment studies are carried out and explains their possible benefits and risks.

NCI's Web site includes a section on clinical trials at http://www.cancer.gov/clinicaltrials. It has general information about clinical trials as well as detailed information about specific ongoing studies of leukemia. Information specialists at 1-800-4-CANCER or at LiveHelp (http://www.cancer.gov/livehelp) can answer questions and provide information about clinical trials.

Made in the USA
Charleston, SC
04 September 2014